Table of Contents

INTRODUCTION 5
CHAPTER ONE 7
What is CBD? 7
    CBD and Your Endocannabinoid System 9
    Health Benefits of CBD 11
Medical uses 13
    Epilepsy 13
    Other uses 14
    Potential interactions 15
Pharmacology 16
    Pharmacodynamics 16
    Pharmacokinetics 17
    Pharmaceutical preparations 17
    Chemistry 18
    Biosynthesis 19
    Food and beverage 19
    Plant sources 21
    Non-psychoactivity 21
Legal status 24
    United Nations 24

Australia 24
Canada 25
European Union 25
Sweden 27
New Zealand 27
United Kingdom 27
United States 29
Switzerland 32
Research 33
The Fundamentals of Cannabidiol 33
Cannabidiol is Not Psychoactive 33
Cannabidiol Can Come From Hemp or Marijuana Plants . 35
Breeders Are Crafting Specialized CBD-Dominant Weed Strains 37
What Does Cannabidiol Actually Do? 39
How Does Cannabidiol Interact With The Body? 40
What CBD Can Really Do—And The Research Backing It Up 42
CBD Can Stop Epileptic Seizures 42
CBD Can Treat Serious Neurological Diseases Like Alzheimer's, Multiple Sclerosis, and Parkinson's 43
CBD Can Relieve Pain 44
CBD Can Fight Cancer 45

CBD Can Reduce Inflammation 46

CBD Can Treat Mood Disorders 46

What Can CBD Do For Recreational Users? 47

The Most Popular CBD Products Available Today 50

The Future Of Cannabidiol: The Future Of Healing?............. 51

CHAPTER TWO 53

How much CBD is in a gummy? 53

Take time to get your dose right.. 53

How to find the best CBD gummies 55

CBD Gummies—What's Real and What's Fake...................... 57

FAQs about CBD gummies 58

Is CBD safe?.. 58

Are CBD gummies legal in the United States? 59

Will I get high from eating CBD gummies? 59

How many CBD gummies should I eat? 59

Will I fail a drug test if I eat CBD gummies?...................... 60

Where can I buy CBD gummies?.. 61

The Differences Between CBD Gummies and CBD Oil.......... 62

CBD Gummies Are The Same As CBD Oil! 63

CBD Gummies Are Different From CBD Oil...................... 65

Increasing Popularity of CBD Gummies 67

How to pick the right CBD gummies 71

Note 74
Review Methodology 75
CHAPTER THREE 78
Pain & CBD 78
Maximum Pain Relief With Hemp CBD Gummies 83
How To Pick the Best Brands of CBD Gummies? 84
What Potency & Dosage of CBD Gummies Works Best at Relieving Pain? 86
How to make CBD Gummies 88
CHAPTER FOUR 89
CONCLUSION 89

INTRODUCTION

Reducing chronic pain and improving your quality of life is possible with CBD gummies. Find out everything you need to know about CBD infused edibles and more, before you shop online. Stop worrying about toxic opioids and OTC medications and start getting the all-natural pain-relief you need today!

Is it possible to reduce your chronic pain by taking CBD gummies? Thousands of people taking CBD say yes! Read on to learn why this non-intoxicating compound is making headlines around the world for it's anti-inflammatory and pain-relieving effects.

Why is CBD being infused into everything from oils to foods, drinks, and even gummy bears? It's because CBD is an all-natural pain-reliever that's absolutely safe and is 100% legal in all 50 states. Find out how CBD works to relieve different types of pain and read about everything you should consider before buying online.

CHAPTER ONE

What is CBD?

An acronym for cannabidiol, it's a type of cannabinoid found in the cannabis. There are over 400 chemical compounds present in the hemp. Out of those 400, around 60 chemicals are totally unique to cannabis including hemp. Cannabidiol is one of those compounds that doctors frequently use for therapeutic intervention. The great thing about CBD is that it carries no psychoactive propertiesunlike THC (tetrahydrocannabinol). That is why you don't get to experience the 'high' associated with THC based products. In fact, CBD counters the effect of THC and helps with withdrawal symptoms. It's also supposed to help with chronic pains, inflammation, headaches, and myriad other health problems. This is the reason CBD is not banned in most places. Patients consume

CBD in a variety of forms like oil, tincture, vapes, wax concentrates, powder, capsule, etc. And, now they can avail its health benefits by consuming it in the form of candy.

Marijuana contains high levels of THC, a psychoactive chemical that's responsible for making you feel "high." CBD sold legally in the United States has less than .03 percent THC, which isn't enough THC to make a rodent high. It's safe for consumption for all ages, and clinical and anecdotal research shows its many health benefits. In fact, the FDA recently approved a CBD-based drug called Epidolex, which is a drug used by children and adults to reduce the frequency and severity of seizures.

CBD is available in many different forms. It can be applied topically through oils and lotions, but it's more common to take it orally through gummies, beverages, or capsules. GBD gummies are probably the most popular because they're convenient and tasty. The sweet, fruity flavors of these gummies remove the earthy taste that many people don't like, making it easier and more enjoyable to eat.

CBD and Your Endocannabinoid System

In a moment, you'll read all about the many health benefits of CBD, but it's useful to first examine how CBD works within your body and to avoid misconceptions. It does not in any way alter your cognitive state, so you don't have to worry about being "out of it" or "high" when you'd rather have your wits about you.

Instead, it works in tandem with your body's endocannabinoid system. This system is responsible for receiving transmissions from the cannabinoids within your body. These signals express sensations like pain and contribute to causing inflammation in the body.

CBD blocks some of the receptors in this system, preventing pain signals from reaching the brain. It works very similarly to non-steroid-anti-inflammatory drugs (NSAID) like ibuprofen, dulling the pain and negative symptoms associated with injuries or stress.

When using CBD gummies, it's important to choose products in which CBD is the main ingredient. The gummies you buy online should be low in THC to eliminate psychoactive properties. Some gummies have more sugar and flavoring in them than they do CBD, which dulls the effectiveness of the drug. When taken in the right dose, CBD typically works quickly and has long-lasting effects.

Health Benefits of CBD

The clinical studies on CBD are minimal, thanks to the controversy surrounding them. Much of the research has been performed on rodents. However, research clinics are becoming more familiar with CBD's potential benefits and are seeking funding to perform human trials to prove the effectiveness in the drug.

Rodent studies as well as countless stories and human experiences have shown extremely positive effects of taking CBD for health and wellness. Some of the most common benefits include:

- Relieved Pain

- Lessened Inflammation

- Cancer Prevention and Delay

- Prevention of Serious Illnesses and Diseases

- Reduced Mental Health Problems

- Relieved Stress

- Better Sleep

Some of the most compelling research points to CBD's ability to minimize anxiety. Those who have suffered from anxiety for their entire lives with little respite report amazing results from using CBD gummies. They report feeling almost instantly calm, and they rave about the convenience of taking gummies at any time without hassle.

CBD is becoming more accepted in the healthcare community thanks to studies that have proven CBD to be an effective supplement for reducing the frequency and severity of seizures for epilepsy patients. The FDA recently approved the first CBD-based drug called Epidolex that's used to treat this disorder with minimal side effects.

Because it has proven so effective in this situation and the side effects are so minimal, many pharmaceutical companies have begun taking interest in CBD as an effective drug. Studies are currently being performed to prove the effectiveness of the supplement when used to treat many of the conditions listed above. It won't be long before the world is well-versed in the empirical benefits of taking CBD.

Medical uses

Epilepsy

There has been little high-quality research into the use of cannabidiol for epilepsy. The limited available evidence primarily focuses on refractory epilepsy in children. While the results of using medical-grade cannabidiol in combination with conventional medication shows some promise, they did not lead to seizures being eliminated, and were associated with some minor adverse effects.

Other uses

Preliminary research on other possible therapeutic uses for cannabidiol include several neurological disorders, but the findings have not been confirmed by sufficient high-quality clinical research to establish such uses in clinical practice.

Side effects

Preliminary research indicates that cannabidiol may reduce adverse effects of THC, particularly those causing intoxication and sedation, but only at high doses. Safety studies of cannabidiol showed it is well-tolerated, but may cause tiredness, diarrhea, or changes in appetite as common adverse effects. Epidiolex documentation lists sleepiness, insomnia and poor quality sleep, decreased appetite, diarrhea, and fatigue.

Potential interactions

Laboratory evidence indicated that cannabidiol may reduce THC clearance, increasing plasma concentrations which may raise THC availability to receptors and enhance its effect in a dose-dependent manner. In vitro, cannabidiol inhibited receptors affecting the activity of voltage-dependent sodium and potassium channels, which may affect neural activity. A small clinical trialreported that CBD partially inhibited the CYP2C-catalyzed hydroxylation of THC to 11-OH-THC. Little is known about potential drug interactions, but CBD-mediates a decrease in clobazam metabolism.

Pharmacology

Pharmacodynamics

Cannabidiol has low affinity for the cannabinoid CB1 and CB2 receptors, although it can act as an antagonist of CB1/CB2 agonists despite this low affinity. Cannabidiol may be an antagonist of GPR55, a G protein-coupled receptor and putative cannabinoid receptor that is expressed in the caudate nucleus and putamen in the brain. It also may act as an inverse agonist of GPR3, GPR6, and GPR12. CBD has been shown to act as a serotonin 5-HT1A receptor partial agonist. It is an allosteric modulator of the μ- and δ-opioid receptors as well. The pharmacological effects of CBD may involve PPARγ agonism and intracellular calcium release.

Pharmacokinetics

The oral bioavailability of CBD is 13 to 19%, while its bioavailability via inhalation is 11 to 45% (mean 31%).The elimination half-life of CBD is 18–32 hours. Cannabidiol is metabolized in the liver as well as in the intestines by CYP2C19 and CYP3A4 enzymes, and UGT1A7, UGT1A9, and UGT2B7 isoforms. CBD may have a wide margin in dosing.

Pharmaceutical preparations

Nabiximols (brand name Sativex) is a patented medicine containing CBD and THC in equal proportions. The drug was approved by Health Canada in 2005 for prescription to treat central neuropathic pain in multiple sclerosis, and in 2007 for cancer related pain. In New Zealand, Sativex is "approved for use as an add-on treatment for symptom improvement in people with moderate to severe spasticity due to multiple sclerosis who have not responded adequately to other anti-spasticity medication."

Epidiolex is an orally administered cannabidiol solution. It was approved in 2018 by the US Food and Drug Administration for treatment of two rare forms of childhood epilepsy, Lennox-Gastaut syndrome and Dravet syndrome.

Chemistry

Cannabidiol is insoluble in water but soluble in organic solvents such as pentane. At room temperature, it is a colorless crystalline solid. In strongly basic media and the presence of air, it is oxidized to a quinone. Under acidic conditions it cyclizes to THC, which also occurs during pyrolysis (smoking). The synthesis of cannabidiol has been accomplished by several research groups.

Biosynthesis

Cannabis produces CBD-carboxylic acid through the same metabolic pathway as THC, until the next to last step, where CBDA synthase performs catalysis instead of THCA synthase.

Food and beverage

Food and beverage products containing CBD were introduced in the United States in 2017.[Hemp seed ingredients which do not naturally contain THC or CBD (but which may be contaminated with trace amounts on the outside during harvesting) were declared by the FDA as GRAS in December 2018. CBD itself has not been declared GRAS, and under U.S. federal law is illegal to sell as a food, dietary supplement, or animal feed. State laws vary considerably as non-medical cannabis and derived products have been legalized in some jurisdictions in the 2010s.

Similar to energy drinks and protein bars which may contain vitamin or herbal additives, food and beverage items can be infused with CBD as an alternative means of ingesting the substance. In the United States, numerous products are marketed as containing CBD, but in reality contain little or none. Some companies marketing CBD-infused food products with claims that are similar to the effects of prescription drugs have received warning letters from the Food and Drug Administration for making unsubstantiated health claims. In February 2019, the New York City Department of Health announced plans to fine restaurants that sell food or drinks containing CBD, beginning in October 2019.

Plant sources

Selective breeding of cannabis plants has expanded and diversified as commercial and therapeutic markets develop. Some growers in the US succeeded in lowering the proportion of CBD-to-THC to accommodate customers who preferred varietals that were more mind-altering due to the higher THC and lower CBD content. In the US, hemp is classified by the federal government as cannabis containing no more than 0.3% THC by dry weight. This classification was established in the 2018 Farm Bill and was refined to include hemp-sourced extracts, cannabinoids, and derivatives in the definition of hemp.

Non-psychoactivity

CBD does not appear to have any psychotropic ("high") effects such as those caused by Δ9-THC in marijuana, but may[specify] have anti-anxiety and anti-psychotic effects. As the legal landscape and understanding about the differences in medical cannabinoids unfolds, experts are working to distinguish "medical marijuana" (with varying degrees of psychotropic effects and deficits in executive function) – from "medical CBD therapies" which would commonly present as having a reduced or non-psychoactive side-effect profile.

Various strains of "medical marijuana" are found to have a significant variation in the ratios of CBD-to-THC, and are known to contain other non-psychotropic cannabinoids. Any psychoactive marijuana, regardless of its CBD content, is derived from the flower (or bud) of the genus Cannabis. As defined by U.S. federal law, non-psychoactive hemp (also commonly-termed industrial hemp), regardless of its CBD content, is any part of the cannabis plant, whether growing or not, containing a Δ-9 tetrahydrocannabinol concentration of no more than 0.3% on a dry-weight basis. Certain standards are required for legal growing, cultivating, and producing the hemp plant. The Colorado Industrial Hemp Program registers growers of industrial hemp and samples crops to verify that the dry-weight THC concentration does not exceed 0.3%.

Legal status

United Nations
Cannabidiol is not scheduled under the Convention on Psychotropic Substances or any other UN drug treaty. In 2018, the World Health Organization recommended that CBD remain unscheduled.

Australia
Prescription medicine (Schedule 4) for therapeutic use containing 2 per cent (2.0%) or less of other cannabinoids commonly found in cannabis (such as Δ9-THC). A schedule 4 drug under the SUSMP is Prescription Only Medicine, or Prescription Animal Remedy – Substances, the use or supply of which should be by or on the order of persons permitted by State or Territory legislation to prescribe and should be available from a pharmacist on prescription.

Following a change in legislation in 2017, CBD was changed from a schedule 9 drug to a schedule 4 drug, meaning that it is legally available in Australia.

Canada

In October 2018, cannabidiol became legal for recreational and medical use.

European Union

In 2019, the European Commission announced that CBD and other cannabinoids would be classified as "novel foods", meaning that CBD products would require authorization under the EU Novel Food Regulation stating: because "this product was not used as a food or food ingredient before 15 May 1997, before it may be placed on the market in the EU as a food or food ingredient, a safety assessment under the Novel Food Regulation is required." The recommendation – applying to CBD extracts, synthesized CBD, and all CBD products, including CBD oil – was scheduled for a final ruling by the European Commission in March 2019. If approved, manufacturers of CBD products would be required to conduct safety tests and prove safe consumption, indicating that CBD products would not be eligible for legal commerce until at least 2021.

Cannabidiol is listed in the EU Cosmetics Ingredient Database (CosIng). However, the listing of an ingredient, assigned with an INCI name, in CosIng does not mean it is to be used in cosmetic products or is approved for such use.

Several industrial hemp varieties can be legally cultivated in Western Europe. A variety such as "Fedora 17" has a cannabinoid profile consistently around 1%, with THC less than 0.3%.

Sweden
CBD is classified as a medical product in Sweden.

New Zealand
In 2017 the government made changes to the regulations so that restrictions would be removed, which meant a doctor was able to prescribe cannabidiol to patients.

The passing of the Misuse of Drugs (Medicinal Cannabis) Amendment Act in December 2018 means cannabidiol is no longer a controlled drug in New Zealand, but is a prescription medicine under the Medicines Act provided the product contains no more than two percent THC of total CBD.

United Kingdom
Cannabidiol, in an oral-mucosal spray formulation combined with delta-9-tetrahydrocannabinol, is a product available (by prescription only until 2017)

for relief of severe spasticity due to multiple sclerosis (where other anti-spasmodicshave not been effective).

Until 2017, products containing cannabidiol marketed for medical purposes were classed as medicines by the UK regulatory body, the Medicines and Healthcare products Regulatory Agency (MHRA) and could not be marketed without regulatory approval for the medical claims. As of 2018, cannabis oil is legal to possess, buy, and sell in the UK, providing the product does not contain more than 0.3% THC and is not advertised as providing a medicinal benefit.

In January 2019, the UK Food Standards Agency indicated it would regard CBD products, including CBD oil, as a novel food in the UK, having no history of use before May 1997, and indicating such products must have authorization and proven safety before being marketed.

United States

As of April 2019, CBD extracted from marijuana remains a Schedule I Controlled Substance, and is not approved as a prescription drug, dietary supplement, or allowed for interstate commerce in the United States. CBD derived from hemp (with 0.3% THC or lower) was delisted as a federally scheduled substance by the 2018 Farm Bill. FDA regulations still apply: hemp CBD is legal to sell as a cosmetics ingredient, but despite a common misconception, because it is an active ingredient in an FDA-approved drug, cannot be sold under federal law as an ingredient in food, dietary supplements, or animal food. It is a common misconception that the legal ability to sell hemp (which may contain CBD) makes CBD legal.

In September 2018, following its approval by the FDA for rare types of childhood epilepsy, Epidiolex was rescheduled (by the Drug Enforcement Administration) as a Schedule V drug to allow for its prescription use. This allows GW Pharmaceuticals to sell Epidiolex, but it does not apply broadly and all other CBD-containing products remain Schedule I drugs. Epidiolex still requires rescheduling in some states before it can be prescribed in those states.

In 2013 a CNN program that featured Charlotte's Web cannabis brought increased attention to the use of CBD in the treatment of seizure disorders. Since then, 16 states have passed laws to allow the use of CBD products with a doctor's recommendation (instead of a prescription) for treatment of certain medical conditions. This is in addition to the 30 states that have passed comprehensive medical cannabis laws, which allow for the use of cannabis products with no restrictions on THC content. Of these 30 states, eight have legalized the use and sale of cannabis products without requirement for a doctor's recommendation.

Some manufacturers ship CBD products nationally, an illegal action which the FDA did not enforce in 2018, with CBD remaining the subject of an FDA investigational new drug evaluation, and is not considered legal as a dietary supplement or food ingredient as of December 2018. Federal illegality has made it difficult historically to conduct research on CBD. CBD is openly sold in head shops and health food stores in some states where such sales have not been explicitly legalized.

The 2014 Farm Bill[82] legalized the sale of "non-viable hemp material" grown within states participating in the Hemp Pilot Program. This legislation defined hemp as cannabis containing less than 0.3% of THC delta-9, grown within the regulatory framework of the Hemp Pilot Program. The 2018 Farm Bill allowed for interstate commerce of hemp derived products, though these products still fall under the purview of the FDA.

Switzerland

While THC remains illegal, CBD is not subject to the Swiss Narcotic Acts because this substance does not produce a comparable psychoactive effect. Cannabis products containing less than 1% THC can be sold and purchased legally.

Research

As of 2016, there was only limited high-quality evidence for cannabidiol having any neurological effect in people.

The Fundamentals of Cannabidiol

Perhaps the only thing more complex than the biochemistry of cannabis is its pharmacology. The ways weed interacts with the human body are exceedingly intricate. And the truth is we don't know as much as we should about those interactions—at least not yet.

Nevertheless, we do know some of the basics. So here's your fundamental fact sheet about Cannabidiol.

Cannabidiol is Not Psychoactive

One of the most crucially important qualities of CBD is its lack of psycho-activity. In layperson's terms, this means that cannabidiol won't get you high.

Unlike THC, the cannabinoid with the legendary power of producing euphoric sensations, Cannabidiol is inert.

So when taken on its own, users experience none of the sensations of being stoned. And this is the single most important property of the cannabinoid from the medical—and legal—perspective.

Cannabidiol is Legal Almost Everywhere

Because CBD doesn't get you high, products that contain only this cannabinoid can skirt the legal ban on marijuana.

Technically speaking, its THC—the cannabinoid that gets you high—which is illicit. When you take a drug test, the aim is to detect THC in your body, not "cannabis." If you possessed weed without any THC in it, technically you wouldn't be in violation of the law. Because "weed" without THC has a different name: hemp. And the rules governing hemp are quite different from the restrictions placed on cannabis.

In fact, every state that has yet to legalize marijuana for medical use has some kind of law allowing people to obtain and use CBD-only (or low-THC) products for medical or therapeutic purposes. And in most cases, that means obtaining Cannabidiol from hemp, rather than cannabis flowers.

In places with legal medical marijuana programs, CBD products are widely available and easy to find.

Cannabidiol Can Come From Hemp or Marijuana Plants

There are two main sources of CBD: hemp plants and marijuana. Where a given product comes from depends on the legal status of marijuana in a particular state.

If medical marijuana is illegal in a given state, THC levels determine whether a CBD product is illicit or not. In most places, the limit is extremely low. We're talking under 1 percent THC, with some states opting for a cap as low as 0.3 percent. In this case, the only source that would work is hemp, and CBD products will, therefore, be hemp-derived.

In other places, limits can be higher. Delaware, for example, allows CBD oil to contain up to 5 percent THC. But that's still not enough to get anyone very high.

Sourcing and legality questions aside, the general consensus has it that CBD derived from marijuana is both more potent and more effective.

Many attribute this phenomenon to the "entourage effect," or the theory that one cannabinoid can do its job better when it works together with its companion cannabinoids. Extracting Cannabidiol from cannabis flowers helps keep these other cannabinoids intact, which is why people prefer it over hemp-derived products.

In other words, the source matters. And the buds of the cannabis plant have a richer and wider complement of cannabinoids compared to hemp leaves. So while we're on the topic, here's a quick rundown of the best CBD-only and CBD-dominant strains of cannabis out there.

Breeders Are Crafting Specialized CBD-Dominant Weed Strains

The demand for medical-grade cannabidiol has spurred breeders and growers to pursue new strain genetics that promote cannabidiol production. These strains don't attempt to eliminate THC. Instead, they increase the ratio of CBD to THC, allowing the effects of cannabidiol to shine through.

- Katelyn Faith: named after the 8-year-old for whom it was created, Katelyn Faith boasts a 34-to-1 cannabidiol to THC ratio, making it one of the most CBD-rich strains in the world.

- Harlequin: A legendary medical strain which weighs in at a 5:2 ratio.

- ACDC: This widely available strain consistently tops 19 percent cannabidiol.

- Remedy: As the name suggests, a potent healing strain with an impressive 15:1 cannabidiol ratio.

- Cannatonic: At a perfect 1:1 ratio of CBD to THC, this strain achieves an optimal ensemble effect for medical patients also seeking the benefits of THC.

- Charlotte's Web: Interestingly, this "strain" isn't marijuana at all. Rather, it's a proprietary hemp plant that produces buds with just the cannabidiol cannabinoid.

What Does Cannabidiol Actually Do?

We've covered the details of what cannabidiol is, its basic properties, and where it comes from. Now, it's time to turn our attention to what this powerful little compound can do.

For good reason, cannabidiol dominates the conversation about the medical applications of cannabis. But that doesn't mean CBD isn't valuable to recreational users. In fact, CBD has some special qualities that can make it an important part of any recreational experience.

How Does Cannabidiol Interact With The Body?

All of the 60-plus cannabinoids unique to the plant genus Cannabis interact with our bodies thanks to a network of neurons called the endocannabinoid system.

The endocannabinoid system runs throughout your body. And it's loaded with receptors that bind to the cannabinoids you introduce to your bloodstream when you consume weed.

And it's the chemical interactions of those bonds that create a wide and largely unknown series of responses in your body.

Without distorting the science too much, you could say that human beings are "hard-wired" for weed. The endocannabinoid system runs deep and touches all of the major systems of the body. And that's why weed can do so many things for us, from altering and regulating moods to stimulating appetites and reducing pain.

And even though cannabidiol has no toxicity for humans—meaning, it doesn't make you intoxicated (i.e. high)—it is highly reactive with the endocannabinoid system.

To put things as simply as possible, CBD makes things happen. When it binds to the endocannabinoid system's receptors, it stimulates all kinds of changes in the body.

Most of those changes are incredibly beneficial, and researchers keep uncovering real and potential medical uses for them.

We won't bog you down with the technical minutiae of each of those changes. Instead, here's a quick overview of the major studies and most promising findings about the medical importance of CBD.

What CBD Can Really Do—And The Research Backing It Up

There's no better way to gain an appreciation of just what cannabidiol can do than taking a look at the exciting research behind it. This overview lists the major medical benefits of CBD, then explains the key studies backing them up.

CBD Can Stop Epileptic Seizures

One of the most important CBD studies ever published was a path-breaking study into the efficacy of using CBD as a treatment for epilepsy.

In 2012, researchers with the British Epilepsy Association published a papercalled "Cannabidiol exerts anticonvulsant effects in animal models of the temporal lobe and partial seizures." Their conclusion? "The evidence strongly supports CBD as a therapeutic candidate for a diverse range of human epilepsies."

CBD Can Treat Serious Neurological Diseases Like Alzheimer's, Multiple Sclerosis, and Parkinson's

Researchers are still trying to figure out the exact mechanisms behind neurodegenerative diseases like Alzheimer's. We know it has to do with a protein pathway, and that's exactly the pathway this 2006 study investigates.

Taking a look down to the molecular level, researchers discovered that CBD can actually protect nerve cells from degenerative diseases. Scientists call this CBD's "neuroprotective effect," and it's one of the most promising aspects of the cannabinoid.

CBD Can Relieve Pain

Medical cannabis is quickly becoming the go-to alternative to dangerous and addictive prescription painkillers, like the opioids that are causing an epidemic of overdose deaths in the United States.

A lot of weed's pain-killing power stems from its psychoactive cannabinoid, THC. But cannabidiol is also a potent pain reliever. 2015 saw the most important study to uncover the pain-relieving effects of CBD. In that study, researchers compared cannabidiol to morphine.

To their surprise, CBD worked well in combination with morphine and counteracted the latter's risky side effects. This means cannabidiol can help treat acute pain conditions, along with more long-term benefits.

CBD Can Fight Cancer

It sounds too good to be true. But indeed, pre-clinical trials have shown that cannabidiol has a powerful anti-tumor effect.

The most important study to reveal these powerful tumor-inhibiting effects came out in 2015. In fact, this study looked at a range of non-psychoactive cannabinoids, including, of course, cannabidiol.

In a landmark for medical cannabis research, this study concluded that "CBD slows the progression of many types of cancer, including breast, lung, prostate and colon cancer."

How that works is pretty incredible. Cannabidiol actually makes it harder for cancer cells to grow. In some cases, this causes an increase in cancer cell death. No wonder stories abound about "miracle" CBD cures that shrink tumors.

CBD Can Reduce Inflammation

Cannabis is widely-valued as a treatment for inflammation. Credit goes to both THC and CBD in that regard, but cannabidiol has some special anti-inflammatory properties of its own.

Specifically, cannabidiol binds with the endocannabinoid system to produce a response that reduces nerve inflammation. This is another of its "neuroprotective" qualities and a major reason why CBD is such an effective treatment for neurological diseases.

CBD Can Treat Mood Disorders

Post Traumatic Stress Disorder (PTSD) affects nearly 8 percent of all American's during their lifetime.

Women are twice as likely as men to suffer from it. Finding an affordable, safe, and reliable treatment for PTSD would profoundly impact the lives of millions of Americans every year.

To that end, a pathbreaking 2013 study found that cannabidiol improved people's abilities to forget their traumatic memories. These findings are incredibly important and could be relevant for figuring out how cannabidiol can treat other anxiety and stress disorders.

What Can CBD Do For Recreational Users?

The topic of treating stress and anxiety sets us up perfectly to pivot to the importance of cannabidiol for recreational marijuana users.

One of the most awesome things about CBD for the recreational crowd is its ability to act as a kind of counterweight to THC. The passive, sustaining Yin to the active, creative Yang of THC if you will.

CBD Can Produce A Smoother, More Balanced High

When recreational users report a negative experience with weed, the issue almost always has to do with feelings of paranoia and anxiety. No doubt, any serious recreational user has been there. Today's weed can be incredibly potentin terms of THC. And that's not even mentioning concentrates.

High doses of THC can and do trigger negative mood alterations. And some people are just more sensitive to THC than others. For both people who accidentally got "too high," and those hyper-sensitive to THC, cannabidiol can help pump the breaks by inhibiting some of the toxicity of THC.

This is a really unique and little-understood mechanism covered under the entourage effect. But if you take a close look at dispensary products, you'll see plenty of strains, edibles, and concentrates that include a healthy dose of CBD in addition to high quantities of THC.

The reason for this is that cannabidiol works like an antidote to THC. It counters some of the stronger, stress-inducing effects of THC, leading to a smoother, more balanced high.

Hence, 1:1 strains or other products with a balanced blend of THC and CBD are super-popular among recreational cannabis consumers.

The Most Popular CBD Products Available Today

CBD Oils

Today, the most popular way to purchase products and consume cannabidiol is as an oil. Remember, though, that CBD oil can come from hemp or from marijuana plants, and quality can vary dramatically.

Health and Beauty Products

Additionally, topical ointments, which allow CBD to be absorbed through the skin, are also tremendously popular. Moisturizers infused with CBD extracts are dominating the health and skin care markets for therapeutic cannabis. As are other CBD-infused products like shampoos, facial cleansers and even deodorant.

Vaporizers

Vaping CBD extracts in the form of wax concentrate is another popular mode of consuming cannabidiol.

Edibles

And finally, there's the old standbys: edibles and tinctures for making CBD-infused foods and beverages.

The Future Of Cannabidiol: The Future Of Healing?

That's the rundown of what cannabidiol is, what it can do for you and the most popular ways to get your hands on it. As you can see, the future holds in store some exciting things for CBD, thanks to its seemingly bottomless promise as an effective and safe medicine.

Capable of fighting back against the most serious diseases, while also gentle enough to be a part of a daily health regimen, cannabidiol is truly one of the most remarkable compounds in the natural world.

And for this reason, cannabidiol (CBD) is driving innovation in the cannabis industry. Who would have guessed that the part of the plant that doesn't get you high become such a major player in today's cannabis revolution?

CHAPTER TWO

How much CBD is in a gummy?

First, it's important that you understand product concentrations.

Concentrations vary from 1 mg CBD per gummy to 25 or 50 mg each. If a bag of gummies has 500mg of CBD in a 30 count bottle, you can get an estimate of the number of milligrams per gummy bear. In this case about 17 mg in each.

Other times you will see brands list the milligrams in a "serving." Often a serving correlates to one CBD gummy.

Take time to get your dose right

Dosing guidelines are limited. The best advice is to start low and work your way up to a dose that is right for you. One online resource suggests 1-6 mg of CBD per 10 lbs of body weight. So a 200-pound man might take 20 to 120 mg of CBD. This could be broken out through the course of a day.

Consider concentration when dosing for different conditions. Dosing for anxiety (regular, lower doses) may be very different from dosing for sleep (single, higher doses). That's not medical advice. It's what we hear from people who use CBD.

Dosing is the #1 question brands get. It's the question we get most often. This point can't be overstated: there is no clear or prescriptive answer.

How your body reacts to CBD is unique. How your body reacts to edibles is especially unique. Also, whether you want to "feel relaxed" or simply take a daily supplement is up to you. A capsule may give your body cannabinoids that steadily absorb into your body over time. A CBD vape you'll feel right away. Oils are closer to vapes in how quickly they work, but they take time to get into your system.

Don't immediately take more. The impact of CBD may be cumulative.

How to find the best CBD gummies

Like most other CBD edibles, gummies are made by breaking down industrial hemp plants and extracting their valuable active compounds. Heat is an important factor in this process, but temperatures that are too hot can degrade the amount of CBD that actually makes it into a gummy. Temperatures should not exceed 200 °F during the creation of CBD-infused gummies, although it's very hard for consumers to find out how a particular product was specifically made. If you're serious about your CBD consumption, contact reputable brands or search their websites to see if they have information about how their CBD gummies are produced.

Other than purchasing from a company that properly heats their CBD, here's what else you can look for when choosing a CBD gummy that's right for you:

• Non-GMO products with organic sugars, flavors, and natural colors

• Third party testing, which provides an accurate description of ingredients

• Clearly stated CBD potency so you know how many milligrams are in each gummy

• Whether the CBD was extracted from hemp or marijuana (each one is a different strain of cannabis, but marijuana has more THC)

CBD Gummies—What's Real and What's Fake

There's a lot of misleading information on the internet that makes it even more confusing to find important details pertaining to CBD products. For example, several different websites claim that CBD gummies will take effect in a certain time frame. Some say it can take up to 2 hours, while others say you won't feel anything from CBD until 4 to 6 hours after consumption. Clearly, there are some discrepancies that need to be addressed.

The real answer is that everyone has a different metabolism, and there is no guarantee that CBD will have a certain effect on you. Generally, you can expect CBD gummies to work faster on an empty stomach than after eating a big meal, but it could take anywhere from half an hour to 3 hours (possibly more) for your endocannabinoid system to absorb all of the CBD.

Once you eat a CBD gummy, it may not always be apparent when it has started to work. CBD doesn't necessarily elicit a particular feeling, instead it reduces unwanted symptoms for a sense of overall well-being. The effects from a CBD gummy can last for hours, but exactly how long will depend on the potency of the product and how quickly your body absorbs the compound.

FAQs about CBD gummies

Is CBD safe?
According to the World Health Organization, CBD "is generally well tolerated, with a good safety profile." You should speak to your doctor about how CBD may interact with any medications you're currently taking.

Are CBD gummies legal in the United States?

In a word, yes, but there can be some confusion depending on where you live. For the majority of the country, it is legal to sell and purchase CBD as long as the THC percentage is less than .3%, and you're at the age of 18 or older.

Will I get high from eating CBD gummies?

No, CBD gummies are different than edibles made from marijuana and they will not get you high. There is little to no THC in these small treats. You may feel a sense of relaxation or notice that your symptoms have been alleviated, but you will not have any psychoactive effects like other THC-heavy edibles.

How many CBD gummies should I eat?

The answer to this question is going to be different for every person, and it will also depend on the type of gummies that you use. If you are new to CBD, start with gummies that have a smaller percentage of CBD, and only take one at a time. You won't feel the effects of CBD until your digestive system has started to break down the gummy. For this reason, it's important that you don't ingest too much CBD at once. It won't start to take effect until some time afterward, and after you eat a gummy there's really no way to undo the digestive process once it has started.

Will I fail a drug test if I eat CBD gummies?

Drug tests are looking for THC, and CBD contains no more than 0.3% of THC. This makes it highly unlikely that you would test positive for marijuana on a drug test. Most CBD is derived from hemp plants rather than marijuana plants, which further decreases the likelihood that THC would affect a drug test.

However, if you consume a massive amount of CBD, there is a chance that trace amounts of THC are present in your urine. This could result in a false positive, even though no amount of CBD produces psychoactive effects like THC. According to the U.S. Drug Test Center, as long as you take less than 2,000 mg of CBD in a day you should be safe.

If you're still worried about a drug test and want to stay on the safe side, you can ensure that you'll pass with THC-free gummies and CBD isolates. These products only contain cannabidiol, rather than other terpenes and cannabinoids from the cannabis plant.

Where can I buy CBD gummies?

It's easy to find CBD hemp products all over the internet, just make sure that you are doing your research before purchasing anything that you intend to eat. Lab test results and accurate ingredient lists are a good place to start. This way you'll know exactly how much CBD is going into your body, along with anything else that was used to make the gummies.

The Differences Between CBD Gummies and CBD Oil

In the large world of Kratom consumers, there are a select few who cross the bridge and enjoy CBD gummies along with their Kratom.

However, there are other people in the Kratom community who have never tried CBD gummies, but are very curious to learn what CBD gummies have to offer. We want to discuss how it can benefit you to include a gummy regiment into your daily routine. Being a consistent Kratom consumer, you probably already understand the importance of plant-based practices in your daily wellness routines.

CBD Gummies Are The Same As CBD Oil!

One of the many questions we get about our CBD products is, "what's the difference between your gummies and your CBD oil?"

It's a fair enough question and we want to make sure you understand the differences between the two so you can make an educated selection today.

First of all, CBD stands for "Cannabidiol", and is one of the most comprehensive compounds in the cannabis plant. Let's get one thing clear, there are hundreds of different cannabinoids, but not all cannabinoids are equal to each other. Customers have responded that our CBD products are very satisfying, bringing calmness, clarity, and great relief to their day.

But, let's get back on track, we are here to discuss the one known as cannabidiol (CBD). The more research scientists perform on cannabidiol, the more evidence they find that could revolutionize the medical industry.

The hemp plant is where both CBD oil and our gummies are harvested from. Hemp is in the Cannabis plant family, and you already know the popular plant harvested from cannabis – marijuana.

However, while cannabidiol can come from both the hemp and marijuana plant, the hemp plant is known for producing CBD because hemp produces high quantities of CBD and low quantities of THC. On the other hand, the marijuana plant is known for its high quantity of THC and low quantity of

CBD. So essentially, in origin, gummies and CBD oil come from the same plant, which is hemp.

Both gummies and oil activate the endocannabinoid system in your body. The chemical marriage that happens during this process is beneficial and valuable to your anatomy. The endocannabinoid system is an almost magical process which runs deep throughout the human body and touches a lot of our main response systems. Scientists are still discovering even more positive reactions when the body interacts with CBD, and what a healthy endocannabinoid system means to you.

CBD Gummies Are Different From CBD Oil

When comparing CBD oil to CBD gummies, there is a difference. I have personally received many emails (this past week) where our community is wondering which of these would be better trying first.

There are many scientific reasons behind why you should buy CBD oil and/or CBD gummies, but you are probably wondering which one would benefit you the most? It's important to know the differences between the two.

Here are the differences:

Our gummies are made from the isolation of the CBD compound. CBD oil is made from every bit of the hemp plant. Let me explain.

When I say CBD gummies are made from isolate, this means it is pure CBD. We use a special process of extraction to isolate the compound so you are getting CBD and CBD only.

On the other hand, our CBD oil is made from the entire hemp plant. This means a certain amount of

THC does come with the oil when it's harvested. In case you're wondering, our CBD oil contains the legal limit of THC (.03%).

Increasing Popularity of CBD Gummies

The CBD product market is exploding across the world. There are numerous new products that are coming to market almost every day in this largely unregulated industry. Unfortunately, this means that there's no shortage of businesses that are trying to cash in on the "CBD craze." This has resulted in ineffective, low-quality CBD gummies that are being sold at inflated prices by fly-by-night companies.

Green Roads CBD gummies are one of the few genuinely trusted sources of CBD products available on the market at the moment. All of the Green Roads raw compounds are third-party lab tested for quality, and the fact that the company tests for potency and purity – and posts the results online – just goes to show that they are night and day ahead of the competition. Green Roads also uses Colorado-certified organic hemp, and is the only company we know of that employs a full-time licensed pharmacist to oversee all product manufacturing.

Another way that Green Roads stands out from its competitors is its return policy: You may return your products for a full refund if you aren't satisfied within 30 days. Many other CBD companies won't allow you to return opened products, or they will offer a partial refund for a shorter period of time. One of the reasons that Green Roads has been so successful is because of this unrivaled, extraordinarily high level of customer service.

Another brand we've personally had success with is Hemp Bombs CBD gummies. Hemp Bombs pride themselves on sourcing and importing only the highest grade organically-certified European hemp. And not only do they adhere to the strict European hemp practices, but they have also set up their own quality control standards, which includes third-party lab testing.

Side Effects of CBD Gummies

While CBD gummies side effects have not been studied in a clinical or laboratory setting, there is some research that has been done on the side effects of CBD in general. According to Very Well Health, CBD may result in things like mood and appetite changes, diarrhea, dizziness, and drowsiness. On a potentially more serious level, some have suggested that CBD oil may affect liver enzyme levels.

While the consumption of CBD gummies seems to have few notable side effects (according to our research of anecdotal evidence), it would still be wise to practice caution as some candies offer potent cannabinoid doses. For example, even though CBD gummies come in small sizes, they can contain as much as 25 mg or more of active compounds – definitely enough to make one drowsy or potentially dizzy.

Also, keep in mind that many of the best CBD gummies are made with corn syrup and processed sugars, so it's important to read the label of any product before consumption – especially if you're a diabetic and/or are particularly concerned with the "nutritional value" of what you're eating.

How to pick the right CBD gummies

Edibles are a mainstay of the cannabis community. They are a discrete and tasty option that many people love. CBD edibles come in many forms, too. There are gummy bears, chocolates, caramels, and hard candies, to name a few. The great thing about CBD gummies, specifically, is that you can achieve a relaxing feeling without the psychoactive effects of a gummy that contains THC.

But the tricky thing about gummies is knowing how much to take. We have said that CBD works differently for everyone, and this is especially true for edibles.

When it comes to edibles, your metabolism is another variable in the equation. CBD gummies take effect when they are digested, and everyone metabolizes food at different rates.

If you digest slowly, a gummy may take a while to work but the relief can linger for a long time. For others, an edible may hit them quickly and dissipate soon. Everyone is different.

Be smart:

Most people are taking CBD to achieve some therapeutic value. People want to empower their endocannabinoid system and achieve more physiological balance. Don't you think the restorative power of CBD is offset if you eat a handful of sugar? Think about how much CBD is in a gummy. If you need to eat a handful of candy to get a proper dose of CBD then you haven't taken a supplement—you've had a snack

The best way to vet a CBD brand is to:

• Look for test results: All brands should post recent, detailed test results on their website.

Because testing is unregulated and irregular, Remedy Review does its own testing. If we have recently tested a product and it passed, you'll see the Remedy Review Seal.

• Call the brands: A brand should stand by its product. Some brands offer full refunds if you're not satisfied. If it's hard to get ahold of a real person at a cannabis brand, move on to another. There's plenty of caring people out there who want to help you get better.

• Do some math: Look closely at price and CBD content on edibles. If you're buying gummy bears that have 1mg of CBD each you might need to eat 20 to feel any relaxation. If you're taking CBD to sleep, you don't want to eat a bag of gummy bears before bed.

To help us compile this buyer's guide we spoke with

- Product managers

- Consumer advocates

- Patients and consumers

The common theme of all our conversations is that buyers need to be careful. You should do your research and try multiple brands. CBD as a market is growing much faster than regulations or oversight. It's up to consumers to protect themselves.

Note

You should consult a professional when making decisions about your health, especially if you have a pre-existing medical condition. You should also know that despite strong anecdotal evidence to support the impact of CBD, clinical trials are limited and these products have not been evaluated by the FDA. We aim to be a measured voice, to help you get good info. But our advice is editorial—not medical. Talk to your doctor.

Review Methodology

People are taking CBD gummies for sleep, pain, and anxiety. They are looking for relief. We believe products with this kind of health potential should be safe and of great quality. We also believe the brands that make edibles should be transparent.

We also understand comparing brands is difficult. That's why we want to point out 6 Core Principles that you can use to easily review CBD oil brands. Use these key differentiators to make simple, personal decisions about what CBD brand is right for you.

These are the 6 things we believe customers should use to compare CBD brands and find the best CBD gummies.

But this information only provides a foundation. We've added an additional layer of scrutiny to the buying process.

Once you narrow your list of brands, consider some other things.

Is the CBD gummy full-spectrum or an isolate? We believe full-spectrum products have greater therapeutic value. Some people talk about the "entourage effect," or multiple cannabinoids working together. Experts we talk to support the idea of whole-plant therapy. Look for brands that believe in full-spectrum or broad-spectrum CBD.

Does this brand operate in a state where marijuana is legal? States that have legalized marijuana have more standardized regulations. The industry in these places has infrastructure and processes in place. States that only allow limited cultivation of industrial hemp simply have less resources to scrutinize product development.

Do I want a brand that does one thing great or has everything I need? Consider product diversity. Some people like to shop brands who have a very narrow expertise. Other people like access to a wide variety of CBD products all in one place. The main thing to look out for is white labeling. Is the company who sells everything accountable for the manufacturing of those products or are they a storefront?

Does this brand have assistance programs and military discounts available? Medicine and supplements are expensive. We like seeing brands who make access to their products easier.

CHAPTER THREE

Pain & CBD

Pain is a subjective experience, meaning what hurts really bad for one person might not be very painful at all for others. Not all pain is created equal either. Some types of pain are harder to treat than others. Many severe chronic pain conditions can be so bad they prevent you from completing even the most basic daily tasks.

If you've ever experienced a bruised knee, bee sting, or even a broken bone then you'd be quite familiar with what's known as acute pain. The sharp sensation of an injury accompanied by redness, swelling, heat, and inflammation identify acute pain.

Maybe you stumped your little toe or have a bad skin burn. A couple little CBD gummies could help reduce the acute pain response and stimulate pain-fighting compounds in your body.

Chronic pain is different than acute pain. It occurs daily and for an extended amount of time. The most common forms of chronic pain include lower back pain, joint pain, and migraines.

It can happen for a number of reasons. It could start with an injury or accident, or it can seemingly develop slowly over time for no apparent reason. Millions suffer from chronic pain conditions daily and for the most part are largely underserved by traditional pharmaceuticals like NSAIDs, opioids, and OTC pain pills.

Pain is one of the most common and popular uses for CBD. Not only does it fight the pain that keeps you from being active, but it can also reduce chronic low-grade inflammation that might be causing the pain to begin with.

Millions are finally getting natural relief with CBD oil gummies for many common types of chronic pain including:

- Migraines & headaches

- Face & neck pain

- Lower-back pain

- Joint, hip, and arthritic pain

- Muscle pain & cramps

- Aches and sore muscles

CBD Gummies & Neuropathic Pain-Relief

We mentioned earlier that not all pain is created equally. Studies show that some types of pain don't respond to opioids and normal pain-relief medications very well. However, studies on CBD and these types of pain have given neuropathy sufferers new hope!

Neuropathic pain refers to pain that stems from the nervous system. Migraines are a good example of one type of neuropathic pain. Other severe conditions that can cause neuropathic pain include:

• Fibromyalgia

• Multiple Sclerosis

• Sexually transmitted diseases

• Viral infections

• & More

This kind of pain comes from damage or injury to the network of nerves that run throughout the body. The nerves connect your brain, gut, muscles, and all of your organs together in a very complex and intricate way.

If your nerves are damaged it could affect many other aspects of your health, such as muscles, cognition, and basic bodily functions. Some nerve damage can never be repaired, such as severe brain damage from a stroke where regions of nerve cells are left without the oxygen-rich blood supply they need to live.

Human and animal studies on CBD and neuropathic pain, as well as countless patient reports, indicate that it works better than opioids at providing relief. Using CBD gummies regularly may even protect your brain and heart in the event of a stroke!

Less pain, better rest, and improved health with CBD gummies mean getting the overall better quality of life you deserve.

Maximum Pain Relief With Hemp CBD Gummies

To get the maximum chronic pain relief possible from CBD gummies you'll need to take them as a daily supplement. This helps to build up concentrations of the compound in your body to help reduce pain-inducing low-grade inflammation.

If you have severe acute pain from an injury, you might need to incorporate other CBD-rich hemp oil products like pain-relief gels and lotions. Serious injuries and health conditions do require medical attention; so don't try to replace your doctor with gummy bears! Okay?

Depending on the severity of your symptoms you might need to just take one hemp gummy or a few of them to start feeling the analgesic effects of CBD. How many CBD gummies you need to take will also depend on other factors such as:

- Potency

- Body weight

- Pain severity

- Genetics & environment

How To Pick the Best Brands of CBD Gummies?

Well, for starters, if the price is too good to be true, it most likely is. Processing and manufacturing high-quality CBD requires very expensive equipment and licensing, on top of the normal costs of running a business.

When it comes to CBD gummies, you'll get what you pay for. It's better to not cheap out on lower quality products that may have questionable extraction methods and hemp sources. The best CBD brands will provide a certificate of analysis

(COA) for all of their products to guarantee purity, consistency, and quality.

The highest-quality CBD extract is produced using CO_2 extraction, the cleanest and safest form of solvent-based processing. Make sure you see those lab results and if the company or brand doesn't provide a COA (certificate of analysis) or tell you their extraction methods then you should proceed swiftly to the nearest exit.

You should also look for where the manufacture sources their hemp. Is it organic hemp from the United States (like ours) or is it imported from overseas? Starting with hemp grown in with clean, sustainable, pesticide free farming is vitality important.

What Potency & Dosage of CBD Gummies Works Best at Relieving Pain?

No two people will feel pain in the same way. Just the same, no two person's pain will respond to CBD the same way. To find the best dosage for you first start by picking a potent, high-quality brand of CBD gummies.

It's generally recommended to begin taking CBD in small dosages, and only increasing after observing its effects. Begin by taking 1 mg. of CBD per 10 pounds of body weight in two servings daily for one week and observe your body's response.

If you feel like you need more CBD then you can safely increase to 2 mg. per 10 pounds of body weight divided into two servings per day. Waiting to increase your dosage helps to prevent using more CBD than is needed and can save you money on pain-relief.

Are you still in pain? It's safe to up your dosage without worrying about overdosing or adverse side effects. Just be sure to do so little by little and observe your response. The third week of treatment, you can use 5 mg. per 10 pounds of body weight divided and taken twice daily.

For example, a 150 lb woman who wants to have less migraine and headache pain could safely start with 7.5 mg divided into two servings daily. Of course, many people find that much higher dosages are needed. For example, it's not uncommon for customers to use 15-25mg's before bed. However, we recommend starting slow.

You can easily find CBD gummies that come with 5-60 gummies per package that range in potencies from 15 mg. to 20 mg. of CBD per gummy and up. That means there are a price and a potency that fits everybody's needs.

How to make CBD Gummies

Want to learn how to make your own CBD infused gummies and other edibles? It's not that hard actually, but you will need some basic tools and kitchen skills.

Also, your homemade CBD gummies are only going to be as effective and potent as the CBD oil or concentrate that you start with.

CHAPTER FOUR

CONCLUSION

The main pain-fighting compound at work in CBD gummies is, of course, Cannabidiol. Cannabidiol works by targeting the body's main regulatory system that controls overall health and wellness, called the endocannabinoid system.

This complex system is able to bring bodily functions and biochemicals back into balance, which can help to reduce overall chronic pain and inflammation. When triggered by CBD, the endocannabinoid system essentially tells pain-receptors to send less "pain messages" to the brain, which lowers how much pain you actually feel.

The presence of CBD in your system can also stimulate the production of the natural pain-fighting compounds produced by your own body. Targeting the endocannabinoid system with CBD can optimize and improve the way that your body perceives and responds to pain and inflammation.

CPSIA information can be obtained
at www.ICGtesting.com
Printed in the USA
FSHW022005031221
86700FS